PLANT-BASED RECIPES FOR DIABETES MANAGEMENT

A Plant-Powered Guide to Delicious & Healthy Diabetes-Friendly Meals.

T. John

COPYRIGHT PAGE

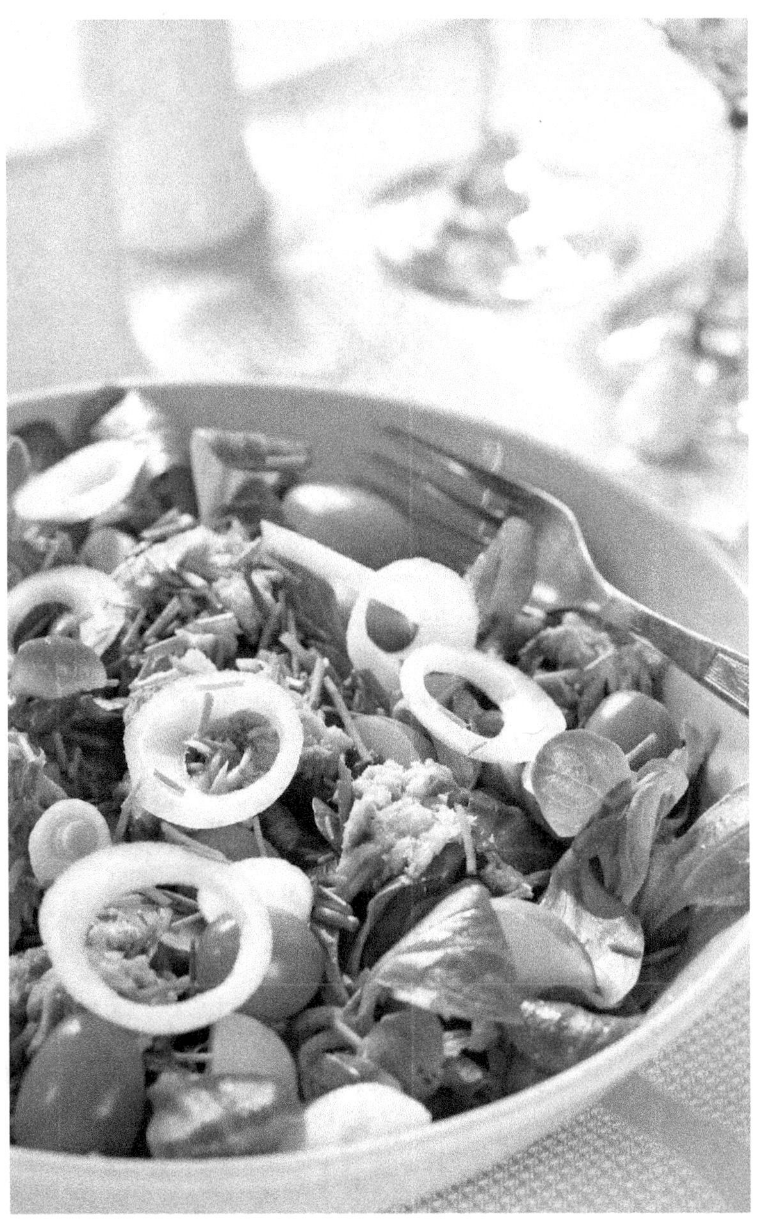

TABLE OF CONTENTS

INTRODUCTION 9

Chapter 1: 30-Day Meal Plan 12

Week 1: 12

Week 2: 14

Week 3: 17

Week 4: 19

Chapter 2: Breakfast Recipes 23

Quinoa Breakfast Bowl 23

Avocado and Tomato Toast 24

Berry and Chia Seed Pudding 25

Oatmeal with Almond Butter and Berries 26

Spinach and Mushroom Tofu Scramble 27

Whole Grain Pancakes with Fruit Compote ... 29

Sweet Potato and Black Bean Breakfast Burrito 30

Vegan Banana Nut Muffins 31

Mediterranean Breakfast Wrap 32

Blueberry Almond Smoothie Bowl 33

Green Tea and Mixed Berry Smoothie 34

Coconut Yogurt Parfait with Granola 35

Chickpea Flour Omelette with Vegetables 36

Peanut Butter Banana Toast 38

Breakfast Quinoa with Almond Milk and Berries 39

Chapter 3: Lunch Recipes....................................40

Lentil and Vegetable Stir-Fry................................... 40

Chickpea and Spinach Salad 41

Quinoa and Black Bean Bowl 43

Vegan Caesar Salad with Tofu................................ 44

Mediterranean Chickpea Wrap................................ 45

Stuffed Bell Peppers with Brown Rice and Black Beans
.... 47

Spaghetti Squash with Tomato and Basil Sauce 48

Kale and Avocado Salad with Lemon-Tahini Dressing 50

Sweet Potato and Lentil Curry 51

Broccoli and Mushroom Quinoa Bowl 53

Black Bean and Corn Salad.................................... 54

Grilled Portobello Mushroom Burger 55

Thai-Inspired Vegetable Spring Rolls........................ 56

Zucchini Noodles with Pesto Sauce 58

Mexican Quinoa Bowl 59

Chapter 4: Dinner Recipes 61

Cauliflower and Chickpea Coconut Curry 61

Eggplant and Lentil Casserole................................. 62

Vegan Stuffed Peppers with Quinoa and Black Beans . 64

Spinach and Mushroom Vegan Lasagna...................... 65

Teriyaki Tofu Stir-Fry... 66

Butternut Squash and Kale Risotto 68

Spicy Black Bean and Sweet Potato Chili 69

Mediterranean Stuffed Portobello Mushrooms 71

Lemon Herb Baked Tempeh 72

Ratatouille with Quinoa 73

Vegan Sloppy Joes with Lentils 75

Thai Basil Eggplant Stir-Fry 76

Quinoa and Vegetable Paella 78

Cabbage and Lentil Rolls 80

Vegan Mushroom and Spinach Enchiladas.................. 81

Chapter 5: Snacks and Appetizers 83

Guacamole with Veggie Sticks 83

Hummus and Whole Grain Pita 84

Roasted Chickpeas with Cumin and Paprika 85

Sliced Apple with Almond Butter................................ 87

Edamame with Sea Salt... 88

Vegan Spinach and Artichoke Dip............................... 89

Carrot and Cucumber Sushi Rolls................................ 90

Stuffed Grape Leaves with Quinoa 91

Avocado and Black Bean Salsa................................... 92

Sweet Potato Fries with Rosemary 93

Vegan Buffalo Cauliflower Bites................................. 95

Caprese Skewers with Cherry Tomatoes and Basil 96

Vegan Spinach and Mushroom Quesadillas................. 97

Zucchini Chips with Garlic and Dill 99

Rice Paper Spring Rolls with Peanut Sauce 100

Chapter 6: Desserts 102

Chocolate Avocado Mousse.. 102

Berry and Almond Crisp 103

Vegan Pumpkin Pie.. 104

Coconut and Berry Parfait... 105

Chia Seed Chocolate Pudding 107

Baked Apples with Cinnamon...................................... 108

Vegan Lemon Blueberry Cheesecake Bars 109

Date and Walnut Energy Bites 110

Avocado Chocolate Truffles 111

Mango and Coconut Sorbet.. 113

Raspberry and Almond Thumbprint Cookies 114

Vegan Carrot Cake with Cashew Frosting................... 115

Banana Walnut Bread... 117

Chocolate-Dipped Strawberries 118

Almond and Coconut Energy Balls............................. 119

Chapter 7: Smoothies 121

Green Power Smoothie with Kale and Pineapple: 121

Berry Blast Smoothie with Mixed Berries: 122

Mango and Spinach Smoothie: 123

Pineapple and Coconut Smoothie: 124

Chocolate Banana Protein Smoothie:........................... 125

Antioxidant-Rich Blueberry Smoothie: 127

Peanut Butter and Banana Smoothie:.......................... 128

Kale and Kiwi Green Smoothie: 129

Citrus Burst Smoothie with Orange and Grapefruit:... 130

Almond Joy Smoothie with Coconut and Almond Milk:
.... 131

Raspberry and Almond Butter Smoothie: 132

Turmeric and Ginger Immune-Boosting Smoothie:.... 134

Tropical Paradise Smoothie with Mango and Papaya: 135

Matcha Green Tea Smoothie:....................................... 136

Avocado and Mint Smoothie: 137

CONCLUSION 139

INTRODUCTION

Forget kale chips and tofu crumbles – plant-based eating for diabetes isn't about deprivation, it's about embracing a vibrant, flavorful, and surprisingly delightful way to nourish your body and manage your blood sugar. Imagine your plate overflowing with sunshine-hued tomatoes, earthy mushrooms, jewel-toned berries, and plump chickpeas glistening with fragrant herbs. This, my friend, is the symphony of a plant-powered plate, and its melody whispers promises of improved health and well-being, especially for those living with diabetes.

But before we dig into the crunchy details, let's dispel some myths. Plant-based doesn't equal rabbit food. Protein isn't an elusive unicorn in this realm. Legumes like lentils and beans, nuts and seeds, and even whole grains like quinoa, all step up to the plate, offering complete protein packages alongside a chorus of fiber, vitamins, and minerals. This fiber symphony plays a starring role in diabetes management, slowing down glucose absorption and keeping blood sugar levels on a smooth, steady groove.

Think of insulin resistance as a traffic jam on the sugar highway. Plant-based eating acts like a magic roundabout, rerouting sugar into your cells more efficiently, reducing the backlog and keeping the traffic flowing smoothly. This improved insulin sensitivity translates to better blood sugar control, potentially reducing the need for medications and mitigating the risk of diabetes complications.

But the benefits go beyond just blood sugar. The rainbow of fruits and vegetables brings a whole orchestra of antioxidants to the party, mopping up free radicals that can damage cells and contribute to inflammation. This inflammation-fighting effect can not only benefit diabetes management but also protect against heart disease, a common companion of diabetes.

And let's not forget the waistline! Plant-based meals tend to be naturally lower in calorie density, meaning you can fill your plate without overloading your belly. This, coupled with the satiating power of fiber, can lead to healthy weight management, another crucial factor in diabetes control.

Now, transitioning to a plant-based approach doesn't require a bulldozer to your pantry. Start small, introduce a few plant-based meals a week, explore the dazzling world of lentils and tofu, and discover the hidden gems of leafy greens and vibrant root vegetables. Remember, it's not about perfection, it's about progress.

This isn't just about food, it's about an empowered journey towards a healthier, happier you. So, grab your fork, embrace the plant-powered revolution, and let your taste buds dance to the rhythm of well-being. Remember, in the culinary concerto of diabetes management, plant-based eating is the melody that can truly harmonize your health.

Chapter 1: 30-Day Meal Plan

Week 1:

Day 1:

- Breakfast: Quinoa Breakfast Bowl
- Lunch: Lentil and Vegetable Stir-Fry
- Dinner: Cauliflower and Chickpea Coconut Curry
- Snack: Guacamole with Veggie Sticks
- Dessert: Chocolate Avocado Mousse

Day 2:

- Breakfast: Avocado and Tomato Toast
- Lunch: Chickpea and Spinach Salad
- Dinner: Eggplant and Lentil Casserole
- Snack: Hummus and Whole Grain Pita
- Dessert: Berry and Almond Crisp

Day 3:

- Breakfast: Berry and Chia Seed Pudding
- Lunch: Quinoa and Black Bean Bowl

- Dinner: Vegan Stuffed Peppers with Quinoa and Black Beans
- Snack: Roasted Chickpeas with Cumin and Paprika
- Dessert: Vegan Pumpkin Pie

Day 4:

- Breakfast: Oatmeal with Almond Butter and Berries
- Lunch: Vegan Caesar Salad with Tofu
- Dinner: Spinach and Mushroom Vegan Lasagna
- Snack: Sliced Apple with Almond Butter
- Dessert: Coconut and Berry Parfait

Day 5:

- Breakfast: Spinach and Mushroom Tofu Scramble
- Lunch: Mediterranean Chickpea Wrap
- Dinner: Teriyaki Tofu Stir-Fry
- Snack: Edamame with Sea Salt
- Dessert: Chia Seed Chocolate Pudding

Day 6:

- Breakfast: Whole Grain Pancakes with Fruit Compote

- Lunch: Stuffed Bell Peppers with Brown Rice and Black Beans
- Dinner: Butternut Squash and Kale Risotto
- Snack: Vegan Spinach and Artichoke Dip
- Dessert: Baked Apples with Cinnamon

Day 7:

- Breakfast: Sweet Potato and Black Bean Breakfast Burrito
- Lunch: Spaghetti Squash with Tomato and Basil Sauce
- Dinner: Spicy Black Bean and Sweet Potato Chili
- Snack: Carrot and Cucumber Sushi Rolls
- Dessert: Vegan Lemon Blueberry Cheesecake Bars

Week 2:

Day 8:

- Breakfast: Vegan Banana Nut Muffins
- Lunch: Kale and Avocado Salad with Lemon-Tahini Dressing
- Dinner: Mediterranean Stuffed Portobello Mushrooms

- Snack: Vegan Spinach and Artichoke Dip
- Dessert: Date and Walnut Energy Bites

Day 9:

- Breakfast: Mediterranean Breakfast Wrap
- Lunch: Sweet Potato and Lentil Curry
- Dinner: Lemon Herb Baked Tempeh
- Snack: Avocado and Black Bean Salsa
- Dessert: Avocado Chocolate Truffles

Day 10:

- Breakfast: Blueberry Almond Smoothie Bowl
- Lunch: Broccoli and Mushroom Quinoa Bowl
- Dinner: Ratatouille with Quinoa
- Snack: Sweet Potato Fries with Rosemary
- Dessert: Mango and Coconut Sorbet

Day 11:

- Breakfast: Green Tea and Mixed Berry Smoothie
- Lunch: Black Bean and Corn Salad
- Dinner: Vegan Sloppy Joes with Lentils
- Snack: Vegan Buffalo Cauliflower Bites

- Dessert: Raspberry and Almond Thumbprint Cookies

Day 12:

- Breakfast: Coconut Yogurt Parfait with Granola
- Lunch: Grilled Portobello Mushroom Burger
- Dinner: Thai Basil Eggplant Stir-Fry
- Snack: Caprese Skewers with Cherry Tomatoes and Basil
- Dessert: Vegan Carrot Cake with Cashew Frosting

Day 13:

- Breakfast: Chickpea Flour Omelette with Vegetables
- Lunch: Thai-Inspired Vegetable Spring Rolls
- Dinner: Quinoa and Vegetable Paella
- Snack: Vegan Spinach and Mushroom Quesadillas
- Dessert: Banana Walnut Bread

Day 14:

- Breakfast: Peanut Butter Banana Toast
- Lunch: Zucchini Noodles with Pesto Sauce
- Dinner: Cabbage and Lentil Rolls

- Snack: Zucchini Chips with Garlic and Dill
- Dessert: Chocolate-Dipped Strawberries

Week 3:

Day 15:

- Breakfast: Breakfast Quinoa with Almond Milk and Berries
- Lunch: Mexican Quinoa Bowl
- Dinner: Vegan Mushroom and Spinach Enchiladas
- Snack: Rice Paper Spring Rolls with Peanut Sauce
- Dessert: Almond and Coconut Energy Balls

Day 16:

- Breakfast: Lentil and Vegetable Stir-Fry
- Lunch: Chickpea and Spinach Salad
- Dinner: Cauliflower and Chickpea Coconut Curry
- Snack: Guacamole with Veggie Sticks
- Dessert: Chocolate Avocado Mousse

Day 17:

- Breakfast: Vegan Caesar Salad with Tofu

- Lunch: Stuffed Bell Peppers with Brown Rice and Black Beans
- Dinner: Eggplant and Lentil Casserole
- Snack: Hummus and Whole Grain Pita
- Dessert: Berry and Almond Crisp

Day 18:

- Breakfast: Quinoa and Black Bean Bowl
- Lunch: Kale and Avocado Salad with Lemon-Tahini Dressing
- Dinner: Spinach and Mushroom Vegan Lasagna
- Snack: Sliced Apple with Almond Butter
- Dessert: Vegan Pumpkin Pie

Day 19:

- Breakfast: Spaghetti Squash with Tomato and Basil Sauce
- Lunch: Mediterranean Chickpea Wrap
- Dinner: Teriyaki Tofu Stir-Fry
- Snack: Edamame with Sea Salt
- Dessert: Coconut and Berry Parfait

Day 20:

- Breakfast: Butternut Squash and Kale Risotto
- Lunch: Sweet Potato and Lentil Curry
- Dinner: Spicy Black Bean and Sweet Potato Chili
- Snack: Vegan Spinach and Artichoke Dip
- Dessert: Chia Seed Chocolate Pudding

Day 21:

- Breakfast: Vegan Stuffed Peppers with Quinoa and Black Beans
- Lunch: Broccoli and Mushroom Quinoa Bowl
- Dinner: Mediterranean Stuffed Portobello Mushrooms
- Snack: Roasted Chickpeas with Cumin and Paprika
- Dessert: Baked Apples with Cinnamon

Week 4:

Day 22:

- Breakfast: Lemon Herb Baked Tempeh
- Lunch: Avocado and Black Bean Salsa
- Dinner: Date and Walnut Energy Bites
- Snack: Avocado Chocolate Truffles

- Dessert: Blueberry Almond Smoothie Bowl

Day 23:

- Breakfast: Green Tea and Mixed Berry Smoothie
- Lunch: Black Bean and Corn Salad
- Dinner: Vegan Sloppy Joes with Lentils
- Snack: Vegan Buffalo Cauliflower Bites
- Dessert: Raspberry and Almond Thumbprint Cookies

Day 24:

- Breakfast: Coconut Yogurt Parfait with Granola
- Lunch: Grilled Portobello Mushroom Burger
- Dinner: Thai Basil Eggplant Stir-Fry
- Snack: Caprese Skewers with Cherry Tomatoes and Basil
- Dessert: Vegan Carrot Cake with Cashew Frosting

Day 25:

- Breakfast: Chickpea Flour Omelette with Vegetables
- Lunch: Thai-Inspired Vegetable Spring Rolls
- Dinner: Quinoa and Vegetable Paella

- Snack: Vegan Spinach and Mushroom Quesadillas
- Dessert: Banana Walnut Bread

Day 26:

- Breakfast: Peanut Butter Banana Toast
- Lunch: Zucchini Noodles with Pesto Sauce
- Dinner: Cabbage and Lentil Rolls
- Snack: Zucchini Chips with Garlic and Dill
- Dessert: Chocolate-Dipped Strawberries

Day 27:

- Breakfast: Breakfast Quinoa with Almond Milk and Berries
- Lunch: Mexican Quinoa Bowl
- Dinner: Vegan Mushroom and Spinach Enchiladas
- Snack: Rice Paper Spring Rolls with Peanut Sauce
- Dessert: Almond and Coconut Energy Balls

Day 28:

- Breakfast: Lentil and Vegetable Stir-Fry
- Lunch: Chickpea and Spinach Salad
- Dinner: Cauliflower and Chickpea Coconut Curry

- Snack: Guacamole with Veggie Sticks
- Dessert: Chocolate Avocado Mousse

Day 29:

- Breakfast: Vegan Caesar Salad with Tofu
- Lunch: Stuffed Bell Peppers with Brown Rice and Black Beans
- Dinner: Eggplant and Lentil Casserole
- Snack: Hummus and Whole Grain Pita
- Dessert: Berry and Almond Crisp

Day 30:

- Breakfast: Quinoa and Black Bean Bowl
- Lunch: Kale and Avocado Salad with Lemon-Tahini Dressing
- Dinner: Spinach and Mushroom Vegan Lasagna
- Snack: Sliced Apple with Almond Butter
- Dessert: Vegan Pumpkin Pie

Chapter 2: Breakfast Recipes

In this chapter, we present 15 breakfast recipes that not only cater to your taste buds but also align with a plant-based lifestyle. From hearty bowls to energizing smoothies, each recipe is crafted to contribute positively to diabetes management.

Quinoa Breakfast Bowl

Ingredients:

- 1 cup cooked quinoa
- 1/2 cup mixed berries (blueberries, strawberries)
- 1 tablespoon chopped almonds
- 1 tablespoon maple syrup
- 1/2 teaspoon cinnamon

Instructions:

1. In a bowl, combine cooked quinoa, mixed berries, and chopped almonds.
2. Drizzle with maple syrup and sprinkle cinnamon.
3. Mix well and enjoy!

Nutrition Information (per serving):

- Calories: 300
- Protein: 8g
- Carbohydrates: 55g
- Fat: 6g
- Fiber: 7g
- Sugar: 12g
- Portion size: 1 bowl

Avocado and Tomato Toast

Ingredients:

- 2 slices whole grain bread
- 1 ripe avocado, mashed
- 1 tomato, sliced
- Salt and pepper to taste
- Optional: red pepper flakes for spice

Instructions:

1. Toast the whole grain bread slices.
2. Spread mashed avocado evenly on each slice.
3. Top with sliced tomatoes and season with salt, pepper, and red pepper flakes if desired.

Nutrition Information (per serving):

- Calories: 250
- Protein: 7g
- Carbohydrates: 25g
- Fat: 15g
- Fiber: 10g
- Sugar: 2g
- Portion size: 2 slices

Berry and Chia Seed Pudding

Ingredients:

- 1/4 cup chia seeds
- 1 cup almond milk
- 1/2 cup mixed berries (raspberries, blackberries, strawberries)
- 1 tablespoon maple syrup
- 1/2 teaspoon vanilla extract

Instructions:

1. Mix chia seeds, almond milk, maple syrup, and vanilla extract in a jar.
2. Refrigerate for at least 4 hours or overnight.

3. Before serving, top with mixed berries.

Nutrition Information (per serving):

- Calories: 180

- Protein: 5g

- Carbohydrates: 20g

- Fat: 9g

- Fiber: 10g

- Sugar: 6g

- Portion size: 1 pudding jar

Oatmeal with Almond Butter and Berries

Ingredients:

- 1/2 cup rolled oats
- 1 cup almond milk
- 1 tablespoon almond butter
- 1/2 cup mixed berries (blueberries, raspberries)
- 1 teaspoon honey (optional)

Instructions:

1. Cook rolled oats with almond milk according to package instructions.
2. Stir in almond butter until well combined.
3. Top with mixed berries and drizzle with honey if desired.

Nutrition Information (per serving):

- Calories: 280
- Protein: 8g
- Carbohydrates: 40g
- Fat: 10g
- Fiber: 7g
- Sugar: 8g
- Portion size: 1 bowl

Spinach and Mushroom Tofu Scramble

Ingredients:

- 1/2 block firm tofu, crumbled
- 1 cup spinach, chopped

- 1/2 cup mushrooms, sliced

- 1 tablespoon nutritional yeast

- Salt and pepper to taste

Instructions:

1. In a pan, sauté spinach and mushrooms until wilted.

2. Add crumbled tofu and nutritional yeast, stirring until heated through.

3. Season with salt and pepper to taste.

Nutrition Information (per serving):

- Calories: 220

- Protein: 18g

- Carbohydrates: 10g

- Fat: 14g

- Fiber: 4g

- Sugar: 2g

- Portion size: 1 serving

Whole Grain Pancakes with Fruit Compote

Ingredients:

- 1 cup whole grain pancake mix
- 3/4 cup water
- 1 cup mixed fruit (berries, sliced banana)
- 1 tablespoon maple syrup

Instructions:

1. Prepare pancake mix with water according to package instructions.
2. Cook pancakes on a griddle.
3. In a saucepan, heat mixed fruit and maple syrup for the compote. Serve over pancakes.

Nutrition Information (per serving):

- Calories: 300
- Protein: 6g
- Carbohydrates: 60g
- Fat: 4g
- Fiber: 8g
- Sugar: 12g

- Portion size: 2 pancakes with compote

Sweet Potato and Black Bean Breakfast Burrito

Ingredients:

- 1 large sweet potato, diced
- 1/2 cup black beans, cooked
- 2 whole grain tortillas
- 1/4 cup salsa
- 1/4 cup guacamole

Instructions:

1. Roast diced sweet potato until tender.
2. Warm tortillas and assemble with sweet potato, black beans, salsa, and guacamole.
3. Roll into burritos and serve.

Nutrition Information (per serving):

- Calories: 320
- Protein: 10g
- Carbohydrates: 60g

- Fat: 8g

- Fiber: 12g

- Sugar: 5g

- Portion size: 1 burrito

Vegan Banana Nut Muffins

Ingredients:

- 2 ripe bananas, mashed

- 1/4 cup coconut oil, melted

- 1/2 cup almond milk

- 2 cups whole wheat flour

- 1/2 cup chopped walnuts

- 1 teaspoon baking soda

Instructions:

1. Preheat the oven to 350°F (175°C) and line a muffin tin.

2. In a bowl, mix mashed bananas, melted coconut oil, and almond milk.

3. Stir in whole wheat flour, chopped walnuts, and baking soda until just combined.

4. Spoon the batter into muffin cups and bake for 20-25 minutes.

Nutrition Information (per serving):

- Calories: 200
- Protein: 5g
- Carbohydrates: 30g
- Fat: 8g
- Fiber: 4g
- Sugar: 6g
- Portion size: 1 muffin

Mediterranean Breakfast Wrap

Ingredients:

- 1 whole grain wrap
- 1/2 cup hummus
- 1/4 cup cherry tomatoes, halved
- 1/4 cup cucumber, sliced
- 2 tablespoons Kalamata olives, sliced
- Fresh parsley, chopped

Instructions:

1. Spread hummus on the wrap.

2. Layer with cherry tomatoes, cucumber, olives, and fresh parsley.

3. Roll into a wrap and slice in half.

Nutrition Information (per serving):

- Calories: 280

- Protein: 8g

- Carbohydrates: 35g

- Fat: 12g

- Fiber: 7g

- Sugar: 3g

- Portion size: 1 wrap

Blueberry Almond Smoothie Bowl

Ingredients:

- 1 cup frozen blueberries

- 1 frozen banana

- 1/2 cup almond milk

- 2 tablespoons almond butter

- Toppings: sliced almonds, fresh blueberries

Instructions:

1. Blend frozen blueberries, frozen banana, almond milk, and almond butter until smooth.
2. Pour into a bowl and top with sliced almonds and fresh blueberries.

Nutrition Information (per serving):

- Calories: 250
- Protein: 7g
- Carbohydrates: 35g
- Fat: 10g
- Fiber: 8g
- Sugar: 15g
- Portion size: 1 bowl

Green Tea and Mixed Berry Smoothie

Ingredients:

- 1 cup mixed berries (strawberries, raspberries, blackberries)
- 1 cup brewed green tea, chilled

- 1/2 cup silken tofu

- 1 tablespoon honey

- Ice cubes

Instructions:

1. Blend mixed berries, green tea, silken tofu, and honey until creamy.

2. Add ice cubes and blend until smooth.

Nutrition Information (per serving):

- Calories: 180

- Protein: 6g

- Carbohydrates: 30g

- Fat: 4g

- Fiber: 6g

- Sugar: 20g

- Portion size: 1 smoothie

Coconut Yogurt Parfait with Granola

Ingredients:

- 1 cup coconut yogurt

- 1/2 cup granola

- 1/2 cup mixed berries (strawberries, blueberries)
- 1 tablespoon shredded coconut

Instructions:

1. In a glass, layer coconut yogurt, granola, and mixed berries.
2. Repeat the layers and top with shredded coconut.

Nutrition Information (per serving):

- Calories: 280
- Protein: 7g
- Carbohydrates: 35g
- Fat: 12g
- Fiber: 6g
- Sugar: 15g
- Portion size: 1 parfait

Chickpea Flour Omelette with Vegetables

Ingredients:

- 1/2 cup chickpea flour

- 1/2 cup water
- 1/4 cup cherry tomatoes, halved
- 1/4 cup bell peppers, diced
- 1/4 cup spinach, chopped
- Salt and pepper to taste

Instructions:

1. Whisk chickpea flour and water together until smooth.
2. Pour into a heated and oiled skillet.
3. Sprinkle tomatoes, bell peppers, and spinach on one half.
4. Fold the other half over the vegetables and cook until set.

Nutrition Information (per serving):

- Calories: 220
- Protein: 12g
- Carbohydrates: 30g
- Fat: 7g
- Fiber: 8g
- Sugar: 5g

- Portion size: 1 omelette

Peanut Butter Banana Toast

Ingredients:

- 2 slices whole grain bread
- 2 tablespoons peanut butter
- 1 banana, sliced
- Drizzle of honey (optional)

Instructions:

1. Toast the whole grain bread slices.
2. Spread peanut butter evenly on each slice.
3. Top with banana slices and drizzle with honey if desired.

Nutrition Information (per serving):

- Calories: 320
- Protein: 8g
- Carbohydrates: 40g
- Fat: 16g
- Fiber: 6g
- Sugar: 15g

- Portion size: 2 slices

Breakfast Quinoa with Almond Milk and Berries

Ingredients:

- 1/2 cup cooked quinoa
- 1/2 cup almond milk
- 1/4 cup mixed berries (blueberries, raspberries)
- 1 tablespoon chopped nuts (almonds, walnuts)

Instructions:

1. In a bowl, combine cooked quinoa and almond milk.
2. Top with mixed berries and chopped nuts.

Nutrition Information (per serving):

- Calories: 180
- Protein: 6g
- Carbohydrates: 25g
- Fat: 6g
- Fiber: 5g
- Sugar: 5g
- Portion size: 1 bowl

Chapter 3: Lunch Recipes

These recipes are crafted with wholesome ingredients, offering a perfect blend of flavors and nutrition. Each dish brings its unique twist to the lunch table, ensuring that your midday meal is not only satisfying but also contributes to your overall well-being.

Lentil and Vegetable Stir-Fry

Ingredients:

- 1 cup lentils, cooked
- 2 cups mixed vegetables (bell peppers, broccoli, carrots)
- 2 cloves garlic, minced
- 1 tablespoon soy sauce
- 1 tablespoon sesame oil
- 1 teaspoon ginger, grated

Instructions:

1. In a pan, heat sesame oil and sauté garlic and ginger.
2. Add mixed vegetables and stir-fry until tender.

3. Incorporate cooked lentils and soy sauce, stirring well.

4. Cook until everything is heated through, and flavors meld.

5. Serve hot.

Nutrition Information (per serving):

- Calories: 300
- Protein: 15g
- Carbohydrates: 45g
- Fat: 8g
- Fiber: 12g
- Sugar: 5g
- Portion Size: 1.5 cups

Chickpea and Spinach Salad

Ingredients:

- 1 can chickpeas, drained and rinsed
- 2 cups fresh spinach leaves
- 1 cup cherry tomatoes, halved
- 1 cucumber, diced
- 1/4 cup red onion, thinly sliced

- 2 tablespoons olive oil
- 1 tablespoon balsamic vinegar

Instructions:

1. Combine chickpeas, spinach, tomatoes, cucumber, and red onion in a bowl.
2. In a separate bowl, whisk together olive oil and balsamic vinegar.
3. Drizzle the dressing over the salad and toss gently.
4. Chill before serving.

Nutrition Information (per serving):

- Calories: 250
- Protein: 10g
- Carbohydrates: 30g
- Fat: 12g
- Fiber: 8g
- Sugar: 5g
- Portion Size: 2 cups

Quinoa and Black Bean Bowl

Ingredients:

- 1 cup quinoa, cooked
- 1 can black beans, drained and rinsed
- 1 cup corn kernels
- 1 red bell pepper, diced
- 1/4 cup cilantro, chopped
- Juice of 1 lime
- Salt and pepper to taste

Instructions:

1. In a bowl, combine cooked quinoa, black beans, corn, red bell pepper, and cilantro.
2. Squeeze lime juice over the mixture and season with salt and pepper.
3. Toss until well combined.
4. Serve as a hearty bowl.

Nutrition Information (per serving):

- Calories: 320
- Protein: 15g
- Carbohydrates: 60g

- Fat: 5g

- Fiber: 12g

- Sugar: 3g

- Portion Size: 1.5 cups

Vegan Caesar Salad with Tofu

Ingredients:

- 1 block extra-firm tofu, pressed and cubed

- 1 head romaine lettuce, chopped

- 1/4 cup nutritional yeast

- 2 tablespoons Dijon mustard

- 1 tablespoon capers, chopped

- 1 clove garlic, minced

- Juice of 1 lemon

- Salt and pepper to taste

- Croutons (optional)

Instructions:

1. In a pan, sauté tofu cubes until golden brown.

2. In a large bowl, combine romaine lettuce, nutritional yeast, mustard, capers, garlic, and sautéed tofu.

3. Squeeze lemon juice over the salad, add salt and pepper, and toss well.

4. Top with croutons if desired.

Nutrition Information (per serving):

- Calories: 280
- Protein: 20g
- Carbohydrates: 15g
- Fat: 15g
- Fiber: 8g
- Sugar: 2g
- Portion Size: 2 cups

Mediterranean Chickpea Wrap

Ingredients:

- 1 can chickpeas, mashed
- 1/2 cup cucumber, diced
- 1/2 cup cherry tomatoes, halved
- 1/4 cup red onion, finely chopped
- 2 tablespoons Kalamata olives, sliced
- 2 tablespoons tahini
- 1 teaspoon dried oregano

- Whole-grain wraps

Instructions:

1. In a bowl, combine mashed chickpeas, cucumber, tomatoes, red onion, and olives.
2. Drizzle with tahini and sprinkle dried oregano, tossing to combine.
3. Spoon the mixture into whole-grain wraps and fold.

Nutrition Information (per serving):

- Calories: 320
- Protein: 12g
- Carbohydrates: 45g
- Fat: 10g
- Fiber: 10g
- Sugar: 5g
- Portion Size: 1 wrap

Stuffed Bell Peppers with Brown Rice and Black Beans

Ingredients:

- 4 bell peppers, halved and seeds removed
- 1 cup brown rice, cooked
- 1 can black beans, drained and rinsed
- 1 cup corn kernels
- 1 cup salsa
- 1 teaspoon cumin
- 1/2 teaspoon chili powder
- Vegan cheese (optional)

Instructions:

1. Preheat oven to 375°F (190°C).
2. In a bowl, mix cooked brown rice, black beans, corn, salsa, cumin, and chili powder.
3. Stuff bell peppers with the mixture and place in a baking dish.
4. Bake for 25-30 minutes until peppers are tender.
5. Optionally, sprinkle with vegan cheese and bake until melted.

Nutrition Information (per serving):

- Calories: 280
- Protein: 10g
- Carbohydrates: 55g
- Fat: 3g
- Fiber: 10g
- Sugar: 5g
- Portion Size: 2 halves

Spaghetti Squash with Tomato and Basil Sauce

Ingredients:

- 1 spaghetti squash, halved and seeds removed
- 2 cups cherry tomatoes, halved
- 2 cloves garlic, minced
- 1/4 cup fresh basil, chopped
- 2 tablespoons olive oil
- Salt and pepper to taste

Instructions:

1. Preheat oven to 400°F (200°C).

2. Roast spaghetti squash halves in the oven for 40-45 minutes.

3. In a pan, sauté garlic in olive oil until fragrant.

4. Add cherry tomatoes and cook until softened.

5. Scrape the spaghetti squash with a fork, creating "noodles."

6. Toss the squash noodles with the tomato and basil sauce.

7. Season with salt and pepper and serve.

Nutrition Information (per serving):

- Calories: 180
- Protein: 3g
- Carbohydrates: 30g
- Fat: 8g
- Fiber: 5g
- Sugar: 10g
- Portion Size: 1 cup

Kale and Avocado Salad with Lemon-Tahini Dressing

Ingredients:

- 4 cups kale, chopped
- 1 avocado, sliced
- 1/4 cup sunflower seeds
- 1/4 cup dried cranberries
- 2 tablespoons tahini
- Juice of 1 lemon
- 1 tablespoon maple syrup
- Salt and pepper to taste

Instructions:

1. In a large bowl, massage kale with lemon juice until tender.
2. Add avocado, sunflower seeds, and dried cranberries.
3. In a small bowl, whisk together tahini, maple syrup, salt, and pepper.
4. Drizzle the dressing over the salad and toss gently.

Nutrition Information (per serving):

- Calories: 250
- Protein: 5g
- Carbohydrates: 30g
- Fat: 15g
- Fiber: 8g
- Sugar: 10g
- Portion Size: 2 cups

Sweet Potato and Lentil Curry

Ingredients:

- 2 sweet potatoes, peeled and diced
- 1 cup dry green lentils, rinsed
- 1 can coconut milk
- 1 onion, finely chopped
- 2 cloves garlic, minced
- 2 tablespoons curry powder
- 1 teaspoon turmeric
- Salt and pepper to taste
- Fresh cilantro for garnish

Instructions:

1. In a large pot, sauté onion and garlic until translucent.
2. Add sweet potatoes, lentils, coconut milk, curry powder, and turmeric.
3. Season with salt and pepper, then simmer until sweet potatoes are tender.
4. Garnish with fresh cilantro before serving.

Nutrition Information (per serving):

- Calories: 350
- Protein: 15g
- Carbohydrates: 45g
- Fat: 12g
- Fiber: 12g
- Sugar: 5g
- Portion Size: 1.5 cups

Broccoli and Mushroom Quinoa Bowl

Ingredients:

- 1 cup quinoa, cooked
- 2 cups broccoli florets
- 1 cup mushrooms, sliced
- 1 tablespoon olive oil
- 2 cloves garlic, minced
- 1 teaspoon soy sauce
- 1/2 teaspoon red pepper flakes (optional)

Instructions:

1. In a pan, sauté garlic in olive oil until fragrant.
2. Add broccoli and mushrooms, cooking until tender.
3. Stir in cooked quinoa and soy sauce.
4. Optionally, add red pepper flakes for a spicy kick.
5. Mix well and serve.

Nutrition Information (per serving):

- Calories: 280
- Protein: 10g
- Carbohydrates: 40g

- Fat: 8g
- Fiber: 8g
- Sugar: 3g
- Portion Size: 1.5 cups

Black Bean and Corn Salad

Ingredients:

- 1 can black beans, drained and rinsed
- 1 cup corn kernels (fresh or thawed if frozen)
- 1 red bell pepper, diced
- 1/4 cup red onion, finely chopped
- 1/4 cup cilantro, chopped
- Juice of 2 limes
- 2 tablespoons olive oil
- Salt and pepper to taste

Instructions:

1. In a bowl, combine black beans, corn, bell pepper, red onion, and cilantro.
2. Whisk together lime juice, olive oil, salt, and pepper in a separate bowl.
3. Pour the dressing over the salad and toss gently.

4. Chill before serving.

Nutrition Information (per serving):

- Calories: 220

- Protein: 8g

- Carbohydrates: 35g

- Fat: 8g

- Fiber: 10g

- Sugar: 5g

- Portion Size: 1.5 cups

Grilled Portobello Mushroom Burger

Ingredients:

- 4 large portobello mushrooms

- 1/4 cup balsamic vinegar

- 2 tablespoons olive oil

- 2 cloves garlic, minced

- 1 teaspoon dried thyme

- Salt and pepper to taste

- Whole-grain burger buns

- Toppings: lettuce, tomato, avocado

Instructions:

1. In a bowl, mix balsamic vinegar, olive oil, garlic, thyme, salt, and pepper.
2. Marinate portobello mushrooms in the mixture for at least 30 minutes.
3. Grill mushrooms for 4-5 minutes on each side.
4. Serve on whole-grain buns with desired toppings.

Nutrition Information (per serving):

- Calories: 280
- Protein: 12g
- Carbohydrates: 40g
- Fat: 10g
- Fiber: 8g
- Sugar: 5g
- Portion Size: 1 burger

Thai-Inspired Vegetable Spring Rolls

Ingredients:

- 8 rice paper wrappers

- 2 cups vermicelli rice noodles, cooked

- 1 cup cucumber, julienned

- 1 cup carrots, julienned

- 1/2 cup fresh mint leaves

- 1/2 cup fresh cilantro leaves

- 1/4 cup peanuts, chopped

- 1/4 cup hoisin sauce

- 2 tablespoons soy sauce

- 1 tablespoon lime juice

Instructions:

1. Soak rice paper wrappers in warm water until pliable.

2. Place a small portion of cooked rice noodles, cucumber, carrots, mint, and cilantro on each wrapper.

3. Sprinkle with chopped peanuts.

4. Drizzle hoisin sauce, soy sauce, and lime juice over the ingredients.

5. Roll tightly and serve.

Nutrition Information (per serving):

- Calories: 220

- Protein: 6g

- Carbohydrates: 35g

- Fat: 8g

- Fiber: 5g

- Sugar: 5g

- Portion Size: 2 rolls

Zucchini Noodles with Pesto Sauce

Ingredients:

- 4 medium zucchinis, spiralized

- 1 cup cherry tomatoes, halved

- 1/2 cup pine nuts

- 2 cups fresh basil leaves

- 1/2 cup nutritional yeast

- 2 cloves garlic

- 1/2 cup olive oil

- Salt and pepper to taste

Instructions:

1. In a food processor, blend basil, pine nuts, nutritional yeast, and garlic.

2. Gradually add olive oil until a smooth pesto sauce forms.

3. Toss zucchini noodles and cherry tomatoes with the pesto.

4. Season with salt and pepper to taste.

Nutrition Information (per serving):

- Calories: 250
- Protein: 8g
- Carbohydrates: 15g
- Fat: 20g
- Fiber: 5g
- Sugar: 5g
- Portion Size: 2 cups

Mexican Quinoa Bowl

Ingredients:

- 1 cup quinoa, cooked
- 1 can black beans, drained and rinsed
- 1 cup corn kernels
- 1 avocado, diced
- 1/2 cup cherry tomatoes, halved

- 1/4 cup red onion, finely chopped
- 1/4 cup fresh cilantro, chopped
- Juice of 1 lime
- 1 teaspoon cumin
- Salt and pepper to taste

Instructions:

1. In a bowl, combine cooked quinoa, black beans, corn, avocado, tomatoes, red onion, and cilantro.
2. Squeeze lime juice over the mixture and sprinkle with cumin, salt, and pepper.
3. Toss until well combined and serve.

Nutrition Information (per serving):

- Calories: 300
- Protein: 12g
- Carbohydrates: 45g
- Fat: 10g
- Fiber: 10g
- Sugar: 5g
- Portion Size: 1.5 cups

Chapter 4: Dinner Recipes

These recipes are thoughtfully curated to not only tantalize your taste buds but also contribute to diabetes management through wholesome, plant-based ingredients. Each dish is crafted to provide a perfect balance of flavors, textures, and nutritional benefits.

Cauliflower and Chickpea Coconut Curry

Ingredients:

- 1 cauliflower, cut into florets
- 1 can chickpeas, drained and rinsed
- 1 can coconut milk
- 1 onion, finely chopped
- 2 cloves garlic, minced
- 1 tablespoon curry powder
- 1 teaspoon turmeric
- Salt and pepper to taste

Instructions:

1. In a large pan, sauté onions and garlic until golden
    brown.
2. Add cauliflower florets and chickpeas, stirring well.
3. Pour in coconut milk and season with curry powder,
    turmeric, salt, and pepper.
4. Simmer until cauliflower is tender.
5. Serve over quinoa or brown rice.

Nutrition Information (per serving):

- Calories: 350
- Protein: 12g
- Carbohydrates: 40g
- Fat: 18g
- Fiber: 10g
- Sugar: 8g
- Portion Size: 1.5 cups

Eggplant and Lentil Casserole

Ingredients:

- 2 eggplants, sliced
- 1 cup dry green lentils, cooked

- 1 can diced tomatoes

- 1 onion, diced

- 3 cloves garlic, minced

- 1 teaspoon cumin

- 1 teaspoon paprika

- Salt and pepper to taste

Instructions:

1. Preheat oven to 375°F (190°C).

2. Sauté onions and garlic until softened.

3. Layer eggplant slices, cooked lentils, and diced tomatoes in a baking dish.

4. Sprinkle with cumin, paprika, salt, and pepper.

5. Bake for 30-35 minutes until eggplant is tender.

Nutrition Information (per serving):

- Calories: 280

- Protein: 15g

- Carbohydrates: 45g

- Fat: 5g

- Fiber: 16g

- Sugar: 8g

- Portion Size: 1.25 cups

Vegan Stuffed Peppers with Quinoa and Black Beans

Ingredients:

- 6 bell peppers, halved
- 1 cup quinoa, cooked
- 1 can black beans, drained and rinsed
- 1 cup corn kernels
- 1 cup diced tomatoes
- 1 teaspoon cumin
- 1 teaspoon chili powder
- Salt and pepper to taste

Instructions:

1. Preheat oven to 350°F (175°C).
2. In a bowl, mix quinoa, black beans, corn, tomatoes, cumin, chili powder, salt, and pepper.
3. Stuff each pepper half with the mixture.
4. Bake for 25-30 minutes until peppers are tender.

Nutrition Information (per serving):

- Calories: 320
- Protein: 14g
- Carbohydrates: 60g
- Fat: 4g
- Fiber: 12g
- Sugar: 8g
- Portion Size: 2 pepper halves

Spinach and Mushroom Vegan Lasagna

Ingredients:

- 9 lasagna noodles, cooked
- 2 cups spinach, chopped
- 2 cups mushrooms, sliced
- 2 cups tomato sauce
- 1 cup vegan ricotta cheese
- 1 teaspoon oregano
- Salt and pepper to taste

Instructions:

1. Preheat oven to 375°F (190°C).

2. In a pan, sauté mushrooms and spinach until cooked.

3. In a baking dish, layer noodles, tomato sauce, sautéed vegetables, and vegan ricotta.

4. Repeat layers, ending with a layer of tomato sauce.

5. Sprinkle with oregano, salt, and pepper.

6. Bake for 30-35 minutes until bubbly.

Nutrition Information (per serving):

- Calories: 280

- Protein: 14g

- Carbohydrates: 45g

- Fat: 6g

- Fiber: 7g

- Sugar: 5g

- Portion Size: 1 square

Teriyaki Tofu Stir-Fry

Ingredients:

- 1 block firm tofu, cubed

- 2 cups broccoli florets

- 1 bell pepper, sliced

- 1 carrot, julienned

- 1 cup snap peas

- 1/4 cup low-sodium teriyaki sauce

- 2 tablespoons sesame oil

- 1 tablespoon ginger, grated

- 2 cloves garlic, minced

Instructions:

1. In a wok, sauté tofu cubes in sesame oil until golden.

2. Add ginger and garlic, stir-frying for 1-2 minutes.

3. Add broccoli, bell pepper, carrot, and snap peas. Stir-fry until vegetables are tender-crisp.

4. Pour teriyaki sauce over the tofu and vegetables. Toss to coat.

5. Serve over brown rice or quinoa.

Nutrition Information (per serving):

- Calories: 320

- Protein: 16g

- Carbohydrates: 35g

- Fat: 14g

- Fiber: 8g

- Sugar: 10g

- Portion Size: 1.5 cups

Butternut Squash and Kale Risotto

Ingredients:

- 2 cups butternut squash, diced

- 1 cup kale, chopped

- 1 1/2 cups Arborio rice

- 1/2 cup dry white wine

- 4 cups vegetable broth, warm

- 1 onion, finely chopped

- 2 cloves garlic, minced

- 1/4 cup nutritional yeast

- Salt and pepper to taste

Instructions:

1. In a large pot, sauté onions and garlic until translucent.

2. Add Arborio rice and cook for 1-2 minutes.

3. Pour in the white wine and stir until absorbed.

4. Gradually add warm vegetable broth, stirring constantly until rice is cooked.

5. Stir in butternut squash, kale, nutritional yeast, salt, and pepper.

6. Cook until squash is tender.

Nutrition Information (per serving):

- Calories: 350
- Protein: 8g
- Carbohydrates: 70g
- Fat: 4g
- Fiber: 6g
- Sugar: 3g
- Portion Size: 1 cup

Spicy Black Bean and Sweet Potato Chili

Ingredients:

- 2 sweet potatoes, diced
- 2 cans black beans, drained and rinsed
- 1 can diced tomatoes

- 1 onion, diced

- 3 cloves garlic, minced

- 2 teaspoons chili powder

- 1 teaspoon cumin

- 1/2 teaspoon cayenne pepper

- Salt and pepper to taste

Instructions:

1. In a large pot, sauté onions and garlic until fragrant.

2. Add sweet potatoes, black beans, diced tomatoes, chili powder, cumin, cayenne pepper, salt, and pepper.

3. Simmer until sweet potatoes are tender.

4. Adjust seasonings to taste.

Nutrition Information (per serving):

- Calories: 300

- Protein: 14g

- Carbohydrates: 55g

- Fat: 2g

- Fiber: 15g

- Sugar: 8g

- Portion Size: 1.5 cups

Mediterranean Stuffed Portobello Mushrooms

Ingredients:

- 4 large Portobello mushrooms
- 1 cup quinoa, cooked
- 1 cup cherry tomatoes, halved
- 1/2 cup Kalamata olives, chopped
- 1/4 cup red onion, finely diced
- 2 tablespoons balsamic vinegar
- 1 tablespoon olive oil
- 1 teaspoon dried oregano
- Salt and pepper to taste

Instructions:

1. Preheat oven to 375°F (190°C).
2. Clean Portobello mushrooms and remove stems.
3. In a bowl, mix quinoa, cherry tomatoes, olives, red onion, balsamic vinegar, olive oil, oregano, salt, and pepper.

4. Stuff each mushroom with the quinoa mixture.

5. Bake for 20-25 minutes until mushrooms are tender.

Nutrition Information (per serving):

- Calories: 250

- Protein: 10g

- Carbohydrates: 40g

- Fat: 6g

- Fiber: 8g

- Sugar: 5g

- Portion Size: 1 stuffed mushroom

Lemon Herb Baked Tempeh

Ingredients:

- 1 package tempeh, sliced

- 1/4 cup lemon juice

- 2 tablespoons olive oil

- 1 tablespoon soy sauce

- 1 teaspoon dried thyme

- 1 teaspoon dried rosemary

- 1 teaspoon garlic powder

- Salt and pepper to taste

Instructions:

1. Preheat oven to 375°F (190°C).

2. In a bowl, whisk together lemon juice, olive oil, soy sauce, thyme, rosemary, garlic powder, salt, and pepper.

3. Marinate tempeh slices in the mixture for 15-20 minutes.

4. Place tempeh on a baking sheet and bake for 20-25 minutes until golden.

Nutrition Information (per serving):

- Calories: 280
- Protein: 18g
- Carbohydrates: 10g
- Fat: 20g
- Fiber: 5g
- Sugar: 2g
- Portion Size: 4 slices

Ratatouille with Quinoa

Ingredients:

- 1 eggplant, diced

- 1 zucchini, diced

- 1 bell pepper, diced

- 1 onion, diced

- 2 cloves garlic, minced

- 1 can diced tomatoes

- 1 teaspoon dried basil

- 1 teaspoon dried thyme

- Salt and pepper to taste

- 1 cup quinoa, cooked

Instructions:

1. In a large pan, sauté onions and garlic until softened.

2. Add eggplant, zucchini, bell pepper, and cook until vegetables are tender.

3. Stir in diced tomatoes, basil, thyme, salt, and pepper.

4. Simmer until flavors meld.

5. Serve over cooked quinoa.

Nutrition Information (per serving):

- Calories: 320

- Protein: 12g

- Carbohydrates: 60g

- Fat: 5g
- Fiber: 12g
- Sugar: 10g
- Portion Size: 1.5 cups

Vegan Sloppy Joes with Lentils

Ingredients:

- 1 cup dry lentils, cooked
- 1 onion, diced
- 1 bell pepper, diced
- 1 can tomato sauce
- 2 tablespoons tomato paste
- 2 tablespoons maple syrup
- 1 tablespoon soy sauce
- 1 teaspoon chili powder
- 1/2 teaspoon smoked paprika
- Salt and pepper to taste
- Whole grain burger buns

Instructions:

1. In a pan, sauté onions and bell peppers until softened.

2. Add cooked lentils, tomato sauce, tomato paste, maple syrup, soy sauce, chili powder, smoked paprika, salt, and pepper.

3. Simmer until flavors meld.

4. Serve the lentil mixture on whole grain burger buns.

Nutrition Information (per serving):

- Calories: 280
- Protein: 15g
- Carbohydrates: 45g
- Fat: 3g
- Fiber: 10g
- Sugar: 12g
- Portion Size: 1 sandwich

Thai Basil Eggplant Stir-Fry

Ingredients:

- 2 eggplants, cubed
- 1 bell pepper, sliced
- 1 cup snap peas
- 1/4 cup fresh basil, chopped
- 3 tablespoons soy sauce

- 1 tablespoon rice vinegar
- 1 tablespoon maple syrup
- 1 tablespoon sesame oil
- 2 cloves garlic, minced
- 1 teaspoon ginger, grated
- Cooked brown rice for serving

Instructions:

1. In a wok, heat sesame oil and sauté garlic and ginger until fragrant.
2. Add eggplants, bell pepper, snap peas, soy sauce, rice vinegar, maple syrup, and stir-fry until vegetables are tender.
3. Stir in fresh basil.
4. Serve over cooked brown rice.

Nutrition Information (per serving):

- Calories: 300
- Protein: 8g
- Carbohydrates: 50g
- Fat: 10g
- Fiber: 12g

- Sugar: 12g

- Portion Size: 1.5 cups

Quinoa and Vegetable Paella

Ingredients:

- 1 cup quinoa, uncooked

- 1 onion, diced

- 2 cloves garlic, minced

- 1 bell pepper, sliced

- 1 cup cherry tomatoes, halved

- 1 cup artichoke hearts, quartered

- 1 cup green beans, trimmed

- 1 teaspoon smoked paprika

- 1 teaspoon turmeric

- 1/2 teaspoon saffron threads (optional)

- 2 cups vegetable broth

- Salt and pepper to taste

- Lemon wedges for serving

Instructions:

1. In a paella pan, sauté onions and garlic until softened.

2. Add bell pepper, cherry tomatoes, artichoke hearts, and green beans. Cook until vegetables are slightly tender.

3. Stir in quinoa, smoked paprika, turmeric, and saffron threads.

4. Pour vegetable broth into the pan. Season with salt and pepper.

5. Simmer until quinoa is cooked and liquid is absorbed.

6. Serve with lemon wedges.

Nutrition Information (per serving):

- Calories: 320
- Protein: 12g
- Carbohydrates: 60g
- Fat: 6g
- Fiber: 10g
- Sugar: 8g
- Portion Size: 1.5 cups

Cabbage and Lentil Rolls

Ingredients:

- 1 head cabbage, leaves separated
- 1 cup dry brown lentils, cooked
- 1 onion, diced
- 2 cloves garlic, minced
- 1 can diced tomatoes
- 1 teaspoon cumin
- 1 teaspoon coriander
- Salt and pepper to taste

Instructions:

1. Blanch cabbage leaves in boiling water until softened. Drain and set aside.
2. In a pan, sauté onions and garlic until golden.
3. Add cooked lentils, diced tomatoes, cumin, coriander, salt, and pepper.
4. Place a spoonful of the lentil mixture onto each cabbage leaf and roll up.
5. Place the rolls in a baking dish and bake for 20-25 minutes.

Nutrition Information (per serving):

- Calories: 280
- Protein: 15g
- Carbohydrates: 45g
- Fat: 2g
- Fiber: 14g
- Sugar: 8g
- Portion Size: 2 rolls

Vegan Mushroom and Spinach Enchiladas

Ingredients:

- 1 package corn tortillas
- 2 cups mushrooms, sliced
- 2 cups spinach, chopped
- 1 can black beans, mashed
- 1 cup enchilada sauce
- 1 teaspoon cumin
- 1 teaspoon chili powder
- 1/2 teaspoon garlic powder
- 1/2 cup vegan cheese, shredded (optional)

Instructions:

1. Preheat oven to 375°F (190°C).

2. In a pan, sauté mushrooms and spinach until cooked.

3. Mix mashed black beans, cumin, chili powder, and garlic powder.

4. Spoon the bean mixture and sautéed vegetables onto each tortilla. Roll up and place in a baking dish.

5. Pour enchilada sauce over the rolled tortillas. Sprinkle with vegan cheese if desired.

6. Bake for 20-25 minutes until heated through.

Nutrition Information (per serving):

- Calories: 300
- Protein: 12g
- Carbohydrates: 50g
- Fat: 8g
- Fiber: 10g
- Sugar: 5g
- Portion Size: 2 enchiladas

Chapter 5: Snacks and Appetizers

These recipes are crafted to be both delicious and nutritious, providing you with a satisfying array of plant-powered options for any occasion. Each recipe is presented with bold creativity, ensuring a delightful experience as you explore the world of plant-based snacks and appetizers.

Guacamole with Veggie Sticks

Ingredients:

- 3 ripe avocados
- 1 small red onion, finely diced
- 2 tomatoes, diced
- 1 clove garlic, minced
- 1 lime, juiced
- Salt and pepper to taste
- Assorted veggie sticks for dipping

Instructions:

1. In a bowl, mash the avocados with a fork.

2. Add the diced onion, tomatoes, minced garlic, and lime juice. Mix well.

3. Season with salt and pepper to taste.

4. Serve with an assortment of veggie sticks.

Nutrition Information (per serving):

- Calories: 150
- Protein: 3g
- Carbohydrates: 10g
- Fat: 12g
- Fiber: 7g
- Sugar: 2g
- Portion Size: 1/2 cup guacamole with veggie sticks

Hummus and Whole Grain Pita

Ingredients:

- 1 can (15 oz) chickpeas, drained and rinsed
- 2 tablespoons tahini
- 2 cloves garlic, minced
- 3 tablespoons olive oil
- 1 lemon, juiced
- Salt and cumin to taste

- Whole grain pita bread, cut into triangles

Instructions:

1. In a food processor, blend chickpeas, tahini, garlic, olive oil, lemon juice, salt, and cumin until smooth.
2. Adjust seasoning to taste.
3. Serve with whole grain pita triangles.

Nutrition Information (per serving):

- Calories: 120
- Protein: 4g
- Carbohydrates: 15g
- Fat: 6g
- Fiber: 3g
- Sugar: 1g
- Portion Size: 1/4 cup hummus with 3 pita triangles

Roasted Chickpeas with Cumin and Paprika

Ingredients:

- 1 can (15 oz) chickpeas, drained and dried

- 1 tablespoon olive oil

- 1 teaspoon ground cumin

- 1 teaspoon paprika

- Salt to taste

Instructions:

1. Preheat oven to 400°F (200°C).

2. Toss chickpeas with olive oil, cumin, paprika, and salt.

3. Spread on a baking sheet and bake for 25-30 minutes or until crispy.

4. Allow to cool before serving.

Nutrition Information (per serving):

- Calories: 160

- Protein: 6g

- Carbohydrates: 22g

- Fat: 5g

- Fiber: 6g

- Sugar: 4g

- Portion Size: 1/2 cup roasted chickpeas

Sliced Apple with Almond Butter

Ingredients:

- 2 apples, thinly sliced
- 4 tablespoons almond butter

Instructions:

1. Arrange apple slices on a plate.
2. Spread almond butter on each apple slice.
3. Enjoy this simple and satisfying snack.

Nutrition Information (per serving):

- Calories: 200
- Protein: 4g
- Carbohydrates: 20g
- Fat: 12g
- Fiber: 5g
- Sugar: 14g
- Portion Size: 1 medium apple with 2 tablespoons almond butter

Edamame with Sea Salt

Ingredients:

- 2 cups edamame, steamed
- Sea salt to taste

Instructions:

1. Steam edamame according to package instructions.
2. Sprinkle with sea salt before serving.
3. Enjoy these protein-packed soybeans.

Nutrition Information (per serving):

- Calories: 120
- Protein: 11g
- Carbohydrates: 9g
- Fat: 5g
- Fiber: 5g
- Sugar: 2g
- Portion Size: 1 cup edamame

Vegan Spinach and Artichoke Dip

Ingredients:

- 1 cup raw cashews, soaked in water for 4 hours
- 1 cup frozen spinach, thawed and drained
- 1 can (14 oz) artichoke hearts, drained and chopped
- 1/4 cup nutritional yeast
- 2 cloves garlic, minced
- 1/2 cup unsweetened almond milk
- Salt and pepper to taste

Instructions:

1. Blend soaked cashews, spinach, artichoke hearts, nutritional yeast, garlic, and almond milk until smooth.
2. Transfer to a saucepan and heat over medium heat until warmed through.
3. Season with salt and pepper.
4. Serve with whole grain crackers or vegetable sticks.

Nutrition Information (per serving):

- Calories: 180
- Protein: 7g

- Carbohydrates: 15g
- Fat: 11g
- Fiber: 5g
- Sugar: 2g
- Portion Size: 1/4 cup dip with crackers or veggies

Carrot and Cucumber Sushi Rolls

Ingredients:

- 2 large carrots, julienned
- 1 cucumber, julienned
- 1 cup cooked quinoa
- 4 nori sheets
- Soy sauce for dipping

Instructions:

1. Place a nori sheet on a bamboo sushi mat.
2. Spread a thin layer of quinoa on the nori, leaving a border at the top.
3. Arrange julienned carrots and cucumber along the bottom edge.
4. Roll tightly and slice into bite-sized pieces.
5. Serve with soy sauce.

Nutrition Information (per serving):

- Calories: 160
- Protein: 5g
- Carbohydrates: 30g
- Fat: 2g
- Fiber: 6g
- Sugar: 2g
- Portion Size: 6 pieces

Stuffed Grape Leaves with Quinoa

Ingredients:

- 1 jar grape leaves, drained
- 1 cup cooked quinoa
- 1/2 cup pine nuts, toasted
- 1/4 cup fresh dill, chopped
- 1 lemon, juiced
- Salt and pepper to taste

Instructions:

1. Mix cooked quinoa, toasted pine nuts, chopped dill, lemon juice, salt, and pepper in a bowl.

2. Place a grape leaf on a flat surface, spoon quinoa mixture onto the center, and fold the sides in.

3. Roll tightly, similar to a burrito.

4. Repeat with remaining grape leaves.

Nutrition Information (per serving):

- Calories: 120
- Protein: 4g
- Carbohydrates: 18g
- Fat: 4g
- Fiber: 3g
- Sugar: 1g
- Portion Size: 4 pieces

Avocado and Black Bean Salsa

Ingredients:

- 2 ripe avocados, diced
- 1 can (15 oz) black beans, rinsed and drained
- 1 cup cherry tomatoes, halved
- 1/4 cup red onion, finely diced
- 1/4 cup fresh cilantro, chopped
- 1 lime, juiced

- Salt and cayenne pepper to taste

Instructions:

1. In a bowl, combine diced avocados, black beans, cherry tomatoes, red onion, and cilantro.
2. Drizzle lime juice over the mixture and gently toss.
3. Season with salt and cayenne pepper to taste.
4. Serve with whole grain tortilla chips.

Nutrition Information (per serving):

- Calories: 180
- Protein: 7g
- Carbohydrates: 20g
- Fat: 10g
- Fiber: 9g
- Sugar: 2g
- Portion Size: 1/2 cup salsa with chips

Sweet Potato Fries with Rosemary

Ingredients:

- 2 large sweet potatoes, cut into fries
- 2 tablespoons olive oil

- 1 tablespoon fresh rosemary, chopped
- Salt and pepper to taste

Instructions:

1. Preheat oven to 425°F (220°C).
2. Toss sweet potato fries with olive oil, rosemary, salt, and pepper.
3. Spread on a baking sheet and bake for 25-30 minutes or until crispy.
4. Serve with a side of vegan aioli.

Nutrition Information (per serving):

- Calories: 150
- Protein: 2g
- Carbohydrates: 30g
- Fat: 4g
- Fiber: 5g
- Sugar: 6g
- Portion Size: 1 cup sweet potato fries

Vegan Buffalo Cauliflower Bites

Ingredients:

- 1 head cauliflower, cut into florets
- 1 cup almond milk
- 1 cup chickpea flour
- 1 teaspoon garlic powder
- 1 teaspoon onion powder
- 1/2 cup buffalo sauce
- Vegan ranch dressing for dipping

Instructions:

1. Preheat oven to 450°F (230°C).
2. In a bowl, whisk almond milk, chickpea flour, garlic powder, and onion powder until smooth.
3. Dip cauliflower florets into the batter, ensuring they are well-coated, and place on a baking sheet.
4. Bake for 20 minutes, turning halfway through.
5. Toss baked cauliflower in buffalo sauce.
6. Serve with vegan ranch dressing.

Nutrition Information (per serving):

- Calories: 120

- Protein: 5g

- Carbohydrates: 18g

- Fat: 4g

- Fiber: 4g

- Sugar: 2g

- Portion Size: 1 cup cauliflower bites

Caprese Skewers with Cherry Tomatoes and Basil

Ingredients:

- Cherry tomatoes

- Vegan mozzarella, cut into cubes

- Fresh basil leaves

- Balsamic glaze for drizzling

Instructions:

1. Thread a cherry tomato, a cube of vegan mozzarella, and a basil leaf onto a toothpick or skewer.

2. Repeat until all ingredients are used.

3. Arrange on a serving platter and drizzle with balsamic glaze before serving.

Nutrition Information (per serving):

- Calories: 90
- Protein: 4g
- Carbohydrates: 5g
- Fat: 6g
- Fiber: 1g
- Sugar: 2g
- Portion Size: 4 skewers

Vegan Spinach and Mushroom Quesadillas

Ingredients:

- 4 whole wheat tortillas
- 2 cups fresh spinach, chopped
- 1 cup mushrooms, sliced
- 1 cup vegan cheese, shredded
- 1 tablespoon olive oil
- Salsa and guacamole for serving

Instructions:

1. In a pan, sauté spinach and mushrooms in olive oil until wilted.
2. Place a tortilla in the pan, add a layer of vegan cheese, and top with the sautéed spinach and mushrooms.
3. Place another tortilla on top and cook until the cheese is melted and tortillas are golden.
4. Repeat with the remaining tortillas.
5. Slice into wedges and serve with salsa and guacamole.

Nutrition Information (per serving):

- Calories: 220
- Protein: 8g
- Carbohydrates: 25g
- Fat: 10g
- Fiber: 5g
- Sugar: 2g
- Portion Size: 1 quesadilla

Zucchini Chips with Garlic and Dill

Ingredients:

- 2 zucchinis, thinly sliced
- 1 tablespoon olive oil
- 1 teaspoon garlic powder
- 1 teaspoon dried dill
- Salt and pepper to taste

Instructions:

1. Preheat oven to 375°F (190°C).
2. Toss zucchini slices with olive oil, garlic powder, dill, salt, and pepper.
3. Arrange on a baking sheet and bake for 20-25 minutes or until crispy.
4. Allow to cool before serving.

Nutrition Information (per serving):

- Calories: 80
- Protein: 2g
- Carbohydrates: 10g
- Fat: 4g
- Fiber: 3g

- Sugar: 4g

- Portion Size: 1 cup zucchini chips

Rice Paper Spring Rolls with Peanut Sauce

Ingredients:

- 8 rice paper wrappers

- 1 cup vermicelli rice noodles, cooked

- 1 cup lettuce, shredded

- 1 cucumber, julienned

- 1 carrot, julienned

- Fresh mint and cilantro leaves

- Peanut sauce for dipping

Instructions:

1. Dip rice paper wrappers in warm water until pliable.

2. Lay flat and fill with rice noodles, lettuce, cucumber, carrot, mint, and cilantro.

3. Roll tightly, folding in the sides, to form a spring roll.

4. Serve with peanut sauce.

Nutrition Information (per serving):

- Calories: 160
- Protein: 3g
- Carbohydrates: 30g
- Fat: 2g
- Fiber: 3g
- Sugar: 4g
- Portion Size: 2 spring rolls

Chapter 6: Desserts

These desserts are not just treats; they are a celebration of flavors, textures, and wholesome ingredients. Each recipe is thoughtfully designed to bring you the joy of dessert without compromising your health.

Chocolate Avocado Mousse

Ingredients:

- 2 ripe avocados
- 1/4 cup cocoa powder
- 1/4 cup maple syrup
- 1 teaspoon vanilla extract
- Pinch of salt

Instructions:

1. In a blender, combine avocados, cocoa powder, maple syrup, vanilla extract, and a pinch of salt.
2. Blend until smooth and creamy.
3. Refrigerate for at least 2 hours before serving.

Nutrition Information (per serving):

- Calories: 180
- Protein: 3g
- Carbohydrates: 20g
- Fat: 12g
- Fiber: 7g
- Sugar: 8g
- Portion size: 1/2 cup

Berry and Almond Crisp

Ingredients:

- 3 cups mixed berries (strawberries, blueberries, raspberries)
- 1 cup almond flour
- 1/2 cup rolled oats
- 1/4 cup maple syrup
- 1/4 cup coconut oil, melted
- 1 teaspoon vanilla extract
- Pinch of salt

Instructions:

1. Preheat oven to 350°F (175°C).

2. In a bowl, mix berries and place them in a baking dish.

3. In another bowl, combine almond flour, oats, maple syrup, melted coconut oil, vanilla extract, and a pinch of salt.

4. Spread the mixture evenly over the berries.

5. Bake for 30-35 minutes or until golden brown.

Nutrition Information (per serving):

- Calories: 220
- Protein: 4g
- Carbohydrates: 25g
- Fat: 13g
- Fiber: 6g
- Sugar: 12g
- Portion size: 1/2 cup

Vegan Pumpkin Pie

Ingredients:

- 1 1/2 cups pumpkin puree
- 1/2 cup coconut milk
- 1/2 cup maple syrup

- 1 teaspoon pumpkin pie spice
- 1 pre-made vegan pie crust

Instructions:

1. Preheat oven to 375°F (190°C).
2. In a bowl, mix pumpkin puree, coconut milk, maple syrup, and pumpkin pie spice.
3. Pour the mixture into the pre-made pie crust.
4. Bake for 40-45 minutes or until the center is set.

Nutrition Information (per serving):

- Calories: 250
- Protein: 3g
- Carbohydrates: 35g
- Fat: 11g
- Fiber: 4g
- Sugar: 18g
- Portion size: 1/8 of pie

Coconut and Berry Parfait

Ingredients:

- 1 cup coconut yogurt

- 1 cup mixed berries (strawberries, blueberries, raspberries)
- 1/4 cup granola
- 2 tablespoons shredded coconut

Instructions:

1. In a glass or bowl, layer coconut yogurt, mixed berries, and granola.
2. Repeat the layers until you reach the top.
3. Sprinkle shredded coconut on the top layer.

Nutrition Information (per serving):

- Calories: 180
- Protein: 5g
- Carbohydrates: 22g
- Fat: 8g
- Fiber: 6g
- Sugar: 12g
- Portion size: 1 cup

Chia Seed Chocolate Pudding

Ingredients:

- 1/4 cup chia seeds
- 1 cup almond milk
- 2 tablespoons cocoa powder
- 2 tablespoons maple syrup
- 1/2 teaspoon vanilla extract

Instructions:

1. In a bowl, whisk together chia seeds, almond milk, cocoa powder, maple syrup, and vanilla extract.
2. Refrigerate for at least 2 hours or overnight, stirring occasionally.
3. Serve chilled.

Nutrition Information (per serving):

- Calories: 160
- Protein: 5g
- Carbohydrates: 18g
- Fat: 8g
- Fiber: 9g
- Sugar: 6g

- Portion size: 1/2 cup

Baked Apples with Cinnamon

Ingredients:

- 4 apples, cored and sliced
- 2 tablespoons maple syrup
- 1 teaspoon ground cinnamon
- 1/4 cup chopped walnuts

Instructions:

1. Preheat oven to 375°F (190°C).
2. In a bowl, toss apple slices with maple syrup and ground cinnamon.
3. Transfer to a baking dish and sprinkle chopped walnuts on top.
4. Bake for 20-25 minutes or until apples are tender.

Nutrition Information (per serving):

- Calories: 120
- Protein: 1g
- Carbohydrates: 28g
- Fat: 2g

- Fiber: 6g

- Sugar: 20g

- Portion size: 1 apple

Vegan Lemon Blueberry Cheesecake Bars

Ingredients:

- 1 1/2 cups cashews, soaked and drained

- 1 cup blueberries

- 1/2 cup coconut oil, melted

- 1/4 cup maple syrup

- Zest and juice of 2 lemons

- 1 teaspoon vanilla extract

- Pinch of salt

- 1 cup almond flour crust (pre-made or homemade)

Instructions:

1. In a blender, combine soaked cashews, blueberries, melted coconut oil, maple syrup, lemon zest, lemon juice, vanilla extract, and a pinch of salt.

2. Blend until smooth.

3. Pour the mixture over the almond flour crust and refrigerate for at least 4 hours or until set.

4. Cut into bars before serving.

Nutrition Information (per serving):

- Calories: 280

- Protein: 5g

- Carbohydrates: 20g

- Fat: 22g

- Fiber: 3g

- Sugar: 10g

- Portion size: 1 bar

Date and Walnut Energy Bites

Ingredients:

- 1 cup dates, pitted

- 1/2 cup walnuts

- 2 tablespoons almond butter

- 1/4 cup shredded coconut

- 1 teaspoon vanilla extract

- Pinch of salt

Instructions:

1. In a food processor, combine dates, walnuts, almond butter, shredded coconut, vanilla extract, and a pinch of salt.
2. Process until the mixture forms a sticky dough.
3. Roll into bite-sized balls.

Nutrition Information (per serving - 2 energy bites):

- Calories: 150
- Protein: 3g
- Carbohydrates: 18g
- Fat: 8g
- Fiber: 3g
- Sugar: 12g
- Portion size: 2 energy bites

Avocado Chocolate Truffles

Ingredients:

- 2 ripe avocados
- 1/4 cup cocoa powder
- 1/4 cup melted dark chocolate
- 2 tablespoons maple syrup

- 1 teaspoon vanilla extract

- Pinch of salt

- 1/4 cup finely chopped nuts (e.g., almonds or hazelnuts) for coating

Instructions:

1. In a bowl, mash avocados and mix with cocoa powder, melted dark chocolate, maple syrup, vanilla extract, and a pinch of salt.
2. Refrigerate the mixture for 1-2 hours until firm.
3. Scoop out small portions and roll them into truffle balls.
4. Roll the truffles in finely chopped nuts for coating.

Nutrition Information (per serving - 2 truffles):

- Calories: 160

- Protein: 3g

- Carbohydrates: 18g

- Fat: 10g

- Fiber: 5g

- Sugar: 10g

- Portion size: 2 truffles

Mango and Coconut Sorbet

Ingredients:

- 3 cups frozen mango chunks
- 1 can (13.5 oz) coconut milk
- 1/4 cup maple syrup
- Juice of 1 lime

Instructions:

1. In a blender, combine frozen mango chunks, coconut milk, maple syrup, and lime juice.
2. Blend until smooth.
3. Transfer the mixture to a shallow dish and freeze for at least 4 hours.
4. Scoop and serve.

Nutrition Information (per serving):

- Calories: 220
- Protein: 2g
- Carbohydrates: 30g
- Fat: 11g
- Fiber: 3g
- Sugar: 22g

- Portion size: 1/2 cup

Raspberry and Almond Thumbprint Cookies

Ingredients:

- 1 cup almond flour
- 1/4 cup coconut oil, melted
- 2 tablespoons maple syrup
- 1/4 cup raspberry jam

Instructions:

1. Preheat oven to 350°F (175°C).
2. In a bowl, mix almond flour, melted coconut oil, and maple syrup.
3. Form small balls of dough and place them on a baking sheet.
4. Make an indentation in the center of each cookie and fill with raspberry jam.
5. Bake for 12-15 minutes or until the edges are golden.

Nutrition Information (per serving - 2 cookies):

- Calories: 180
- Protein: 4g
- Carbohydrates: 15g
- Fat: 12g
- Fiber: 2g
- Sugar: 9g
- Portion size: 2 cookies

Vegan Carrot Cake with Cashew Frosting

Ingredients:

- 2 cups grated carrots
- 1 1/2 cups whole wheat flour
- 1/2 cup coconut oil, melted
- 1/2 cup maple syrup
- 1/2 cup crushed pineapple, drained
- 1/4 cup chopped walnuts
- 1 teaspoon baking powder
- 1/2 teaspoon cinnamon
- 1/4 teaspoon nutmeg

- Pinch of salt

Instructions:

1. Preheat oven to 350°F (175°C).

2. In a bowl, mix grated carrots, whole wheat flour, melted coconut oil, maple syrup, crushed pineapple, chopped walnuts, baking powder, cinnamon, nutmeg, and a pinch of salt.

3. Pour the batter into a greased baking pan.

4. Bake for 30-35 minutes or until a toothpick comes out clean.

Nutrition Information (per serving):

- Calories: 220
- Protein: 5g
- Carbohydrates: 25g
- Fat: 12g
- Fiber: 4g
- Sugar: 12g
- Portion size: 1/8 of cake

Banana Walnut Bread

Ingredients:

- 2 ripe bananas, mashed
- 1/2 cup coconut sugar
- 1/4 cup coconut oil, melted
- 1/4 cup almond milk
- 1 teaspoon vanilla extract
- 1 1/2 cups whole wheat flour
- 1/2 cup chopped walnuts
- 1 teaspoon baking soda
- 1/2 teaspoon cinnamon
- Pinch of salt

Instructions:

1. Preheat oven to 350°F (175°C).
2. In a bowl, mix mashed bananas, coconut sugar, melted coconut oil, almond milk, and vanilla extract.
3. In another bowl, combine whole wheat flour, chopped walnuts, baking soda, cinnamon, and a pinch of salt.
4. Combine wet and dry ingredients and mix until just combined.

5. Pour the batter into a greased loaf pan.

6. Bake for 50-60 minutes or until a toothpick comes
    out clean.

Nutrition Information (per serving - 1 slice):

- Calories: 180

- Protein: 4g

- Carbohydrates: 22g

- Fat: 9g

- Fiber: 3g

- Sugar: 10g

- Portion size: 1 slice

Chocolate-Dipped Strawberries

Ingredients:

- 1 cup strawberries, washed and dried
- 1/2 cup dark chocolate, melted

Instructions:

1. Dip each strawberry into melted dark chocolate,
    covering about half of the strawberry.

2. Place on a parchment-lined tray.

3. Allow the chocolate to set in the refrigerator for at least 30 minutes.

Nutrition Information (per serving - 4 strawberries):

- Calories: 120
- Protein: 2g
- Carbohydrates: 15g
- Fat: 7g
- Fiber: 4g
- Sugar: 8g
- Portion size: 4 strawberries

Almond and Coconut Energy Balls

Ingredients:

- 1 cup almonds
- 1/2 cup shredded coconut
- 1/4 cup dates, pitted
- 2 tablespoons almond butter
- 1 tablespoon coconut oil, melted
- 1 teaspoon vanilla extract
- Pinch of salt

Instructions:

1. In a food processor, combine almonds, shredded coconut, dates, almond butter, melted coconut oil, vanilla extract, and a pinch of salt.
2. Process until the mixture forms a sticky dough.
3. Roll into bite-sized balls.

Nutrition Information (per serving - 2 energy balls):

- Calories: 150
- Protein: 4g
- Carbohydrates: 12g
- Fat: 10g
- Fiber: 4g
- Sugar: 6g
- Portion size: 2 energy balls

Chapter 7: Smoothies

These smoothie recipes are not just a delightful treat but also a powerhouse of nutrients. Packed with a variety of fruits, greens, and plant-based proteins, these smoothies are perfect for a refreshing boost any time of the day.

Green Power Smoothie with Kale and Pineapple:

Ingredients:

- 1 cup kale leaves, stems removed
- 1/2 cup pineapple chunks
- 1/2 banana
- 1 cup almond milk
- Ice cubes (optional)

Instructions:

1. Blend kale, pineapple, banana, and almond milk until smooth.
2. Add ice cubes if desired and blend again.

3. Pour into a glass, and enjoy the refreshing green goodness!

Nutrition Information (per serving):

- Calories: 150
- Protein: 5g
- Carbohydrates: 30g
- Fat: 3g
- Fiber: 6g
- Sugar: 18g
- Portion Size: 1 serving

Berry Blast Smoothie with Mixed Berries:

Ingredients:

- 1/2 cup strawberries
- 1/2 cup blueberries
- 1/2 cup raspberries
- 1 cup spinach
- 1 cup water or coconut water

Instructions:

1. Combine strawberries, blueberries, raspberries, spinach, and water in a blender.
2. Blend until smooth.
3. Pour into a glass, and savor the berrylicious goodness!

Nutrition Information (per serving):

- Calories: 120
- Protein: 3g
- Carbohydrates: 25g
- Fat: 1g
- Fiber: 8g
- Sugar: 15g
- Portion Size: 1 serving

Mango and Spinach Smoothie:

Ingredients:

- 1 cup mango chunks
- 1 cup fresh spinach
- 1/2 banana
- 1/2 cup coconut water

- Ice cubes (optional)

Instructions:

1. Blend mango, spinach, banana, and coconut water until smooth.
2. Add ice cubes if desired and blend again.
3. Pour into a glass, and relish the tropical fusion!

Nutrition Information (per serving):

- Calories: 130
- Protein: 4g
- Carbohydrates: 28g
- Fat: 1g
- Fiber: 5g
- Sugar: 20g
- Portion Size: 1 serving

Pineapple and Coconut Smoothie:

Ingredients:

- 1 cup pineapple chunks
- 1/2 cup coconut milk
- 1/2 cup Greek yogurt (or plant-based alternative)

- 1 tablespoon chia seeds
- Ice cubes (optional)

Instructions:

1. Blend pineapple, coconut milk, Greek yogurt, and chia seeds until smooth.
2. Add ice cubes if desired and blend again.
3. Pour into a glass, and transport your taste buds to a tropical paradise!

Nutrition Information (per serving):

- Calories: 180
- Protein: 6g
- Carbohydrates: 25g
- Fat: 8g
- Fiber: 5g
- Sugar: 15g
- Portion Size: 1 serving

Chocolate Banana Protein Smoothie:

Ingredients:

- 1 banana

- 2 tablespoons chocolate protein powder

- 1 tablespoon almond butter

- 1 cup almond milk

- Ice cubes (optional)

Instructions:

1. Blend banana, chocolate protein powder, almond butter, and almond milk until smooth.

2. Add ice cubes if desired and blend again.

3. Pour into a glass, and enjoy this protein-packed chocolaty delight!

Nutrition Information (per serving):

- Calories: 220

- Protein: 15g

- Carbohydrates: 30g

- Fat: 8g

- Fiber: 6g

- Sugar: 15g

- Portion Size: 1 serving

Antioxidant-Rich Blueberry Smoothie:

Ingredients:

- 1 cup blueberries
- 1/2 cup kale leaves
- 1/2 cup Greek yogurt (or plant-based alternative)
- 1 tablespoon flaxseeds
- 1 cup water or almond milk

Instructions:

1. Blend blueberries, kale, Greek yogurt, flaxseeds, and water/almond milk until smooth.
2. Pour into a glass, and indulge in the antioxidant goodness!

Nutrition Information (per serving):

- Calories: 140
- Protein: 5g
- Carbohydrates: 25g
- Fat: 4g
- Fiber: 8g
- Sugar: 15g

- Portion Size: 1 serving

Peanut Butter and Banana Smoothie:

Ingredients:

- 1 banana
- 2 tablespoons peanut butter
- 1 cup almond milk
- 1 tablespoon honey (optional)
- Ice cubes (optional)

Instructions:

1. Blend banana, peanut butter, almond milk, and honey until smooth.
2. Add ice cubes if desired and blend again.
3. Pour into a glass, and relish the classic combo of peanut butter and banana!

Nutrition Information (per serving):

- Calories: 250
- Protein: 8g

- Carbohydrates: 30g

- Fat: 12g

- Fiber: 5g

- Sugar: 15g

- Portion Size: 1 serving

Kale and Kiwi Green Smoothie:

Ingredients:

- 1 cup kale leaves

- 2 kiwis, peeled and sliced

- 1/2 cup cucumber, sliced

- 1/2 lemon, juiced

- 1 cup coconut water

Instructions:

1. Blend kale, kiwi, cucumber, lemon juice, and coconut water until smooth.

2. Pour into a glass, and experience the refreshing green burst!

Nutrition Information (per serving):

- Calories: 120

- Protein: 4g

- Carbohydrates: 28g

- Fat: 1g

- Fiber: 7g

- Sugar: 15g

- Portion Size: 1 serving

Citrus Burst Smoothie with Orange and Grapefruit:

Ingredients:

- 1 orange, peeled and segmented

- 1/2 grapefruit, peeled and segmented

- 1/2 cup mango chunks

- 1 cup coconut water

- Ice cubes (optional)

Instructions:

1. Blend orange, grapefruit, mango, and coconut water until smooth.

2. Add ice cubes if desired and blend again.

3. Pour into a glass, and enjoy the zesty citrus explosion!

Nutrition Information (per serving):

- Calories: 140
- Protein: 3g
- Carbohydrates: 30g
- Fat: 1g
- Fiber: 6g
- Sugar: 18g
- Portion Size: 1 serving

Almond Joy Smoothie with Coconut and Almond Milk:

Ingredients:

- 1/2 cup shredded coconut
- 2 tablespoons almond butter
- 1 banana
- 1 cup almond milk
- Ice cubes (optional)

Instructions:

1. Blend shredded coconut, almond butter, banana, and almond milk until smooth.

2. Add ice cubes if desired and blend again.

3. Pour into a glass, and savor the delightful taste of an Almond Joy in a glass!

Nutrition Information (per serving):

- Calories: 280
- Protein: 7g
- Carbohydrates: 25g
- Fat: 18g
- Fiber: 6g
- Sugar: 15g
- Portion Size: 1 serving

Raspberry and Almond Butter Smoothie:

Ingredients:

- 1 cup raspberries
- 2 tablespoons almond butter

- 1/2 cup Greek yogurt (or plant-based alternative)
- 1 tablespoon chia seeds
- 1 cup water or coconut water

Instructions:

1. Blend raspberries, almond butter, Greek yogurt, chia seeds, and water/coconut water until smooth.
2. Pour into a glass, and relish the rich and nutty raspberry goodness!

Nutrition Information (per serving):

- Calories: 200
- Protein: 6g
- Carbohydrates: 25g
- Fat: 10g
- Fiber: 8g
- Sugar: 15g
- Portion Size: 1 serving

Turmeric and Ginger Immune-Boosting Smoothie:

Ingredients:

- 1/2 teaspoon turmeric powder
- 1/2 teaspoon grated ginger
- 1 cup pineapple chunks
- 1/2 cup mango chunks
- 1 cup coconut water

Instructions:

1. Blend turmeric powder, grated ginger, pineapple, mango, and coconut water until smooth.
2. Pour into a glass, and enjoy this immune-boosting elixir!

Nutrition Information (per serving):

- Calories: 120
- Protein: 2g
- Carbohydrates: 28g
- Fat: 1g
- Fiber: 5g
- Sugar: 18g

- Portion Size: 1 serving

Tropical Paradise Smoothie with Mango and Papaya:

Ingredients:

- 1 cup mango chunks
- 1/2 cup papaya chunks
- 1/2 banana
- 1 cup coconut water
- Ice cubes (optional)

Instructions:

1. Blend mango, papaya, banana, and coconut water until smooth.
2. Add ice cubes if desired and blend again.
3. Pour into a glass, and transport yourself to a tropical paradise with every sip!

Nutrition Information (per serving):

- Calories: 140
- Protein: 3g

- Carbohydrates: 32g

- Fat: 1g

- Fiber: 6g

- Sugar: 20g

- Portion Size: 1 serving

Matcha Green Tea Smoothie:

Ingredients:

- 1 teaspoon matcha green tea powder

- 1/2 banana

- 1 cup almond milk

- 1 tablespoon honey (optional)

- Ice cubes (optional)

Instructions:

1. Blend matcha green tea powder, banana, almond milk, and honey until smooth.

2. Add ice cubes if desired and blend again.

3. Pour into a glass, and relish the unique and energizing flavor of matcha!

Nutrition Information (per serving):

- Calories: 130
- Protein: 3g
- Carbohydrates: 25g
- Fat: 4g
- Fiber: 5g
- Sugar: 15g
- Portion Size: 1 serving

Avocado and Mint Smoothie:

Ingredients:

- 1/2 avocado
- Handful of fresh mint leaves
- 1/2 cup pineapple chunks
- 1 cup coconut water
- Ice cubes (optional)

Instructions:

1. Blend avocado, mint leaves, pineapple, and coconut water until smooth.
2. Add ice cubes if desired and blend again.

3. Pour into a glass, and enjoy the creamy and refreshing blend of avocado and mint!

Nutrition Information (per serving):

- Calories: 160
- Protein: 3g
- Carbohydrates: 30g
- Fat: 7g
- Fiber: 8g
- Sugar: 18g
- Portion Size: 1 serving

CONCLUSION

In the final chapters of "Plant-Based Recipes for Diabetes Management," we've embarked on a journey that goes beyond the realm of mere culinary exploration. This guide is not just a collection of recipes; it's a testament to the power of mindful, plant-centric choices in crafting a healthful and flavorsome lifestyle.

As we conclude this culinary odyssey, it's evident that embracing a plant-based diet isn't merely a prescription for managing diabetes; it's a celebration of vibrant tastes, textures, and nourishment. The carefully curated 30-day meal plan serves as a compass, guiding you through the rich landscape of breakfasts, lunches, dinners, snacks, desserts, and invigorating smoothies, each dish meticulously designed to foster well-being without compromising on indulgence.

Beyond the delectable recipes, this book is an invitation to transform the kitchen into a sanctuary of health. It's a call to appreciate the alchemy of ingredients that not only satiate the palate but also support a diabetes-friendly lifestyle. The intricate dance of flavors, colors, and aromas in each dish symbolizes the harmony achievable through conscious eating choices.

In the realm of plant-based cuisine, every recipe is a brushstroke on the canvas of well-being. It's about savoring the symphony of nature's bounty while caring for your body. The 30-day meal plan isn't just a guide; it's a blueprint for a sustainable and enjoyable lifestyle shift, fostering a profound connection between the food we consume and the vitality we cultivate.

So, as you embark on this culinary expedition, may each bite be a mindful step towards balanced nutrition, and may each meal be a celebration of health and flavor. Let the pages of this book serve as a constant companion on your journey to a more vibrant and diabetes-conscious life. May your kitchen become a haven of wellness, and may the joy of plant-based eating be your daily feast. Cheers to a life well-nourished and abundantly flavorful!

www.ingramcontent.com/pod-product-compliance
Lightning Source LLC
Chambersburg PA
CBHW070950260726
48661CB00003B/1218